S0-ASI-857

Fred Endres

Maxims of Proximity

Fred Endres

Maxims of Proximity

Impulses for a Fulfilled Life

Translated by
Nikolai Endres

edition fisher USA
R. G. Fischer Publishers

© 2003 by Fred Endres. All rights reserved.

No part of this book may be reproduced, stored in a retrieval system, or transmitted by any means, electronic, mechanical, photocopying, recording, or otherwise, without written permission from the author.

ISBN: 1-4107-6558-X (e-book)
ISBN: 1-4107-6559-8 (Paperback)

This book is printed on acid free paper.

1stBooks – rev. 08/08/03

Table of Contents

Author's Preface

My dear fellow human beings in search of proximity,

A book must be the axe for the frozen sea in us. With this quotation by Franz Kafka, I feel inspired to try to cope with the deficits that have been plaguing me for five decades. As long as I work on these shortcomings with my mind only, I miss love. I have to liberate myself from traditional behaviors that make me sick and stereotypes that my (self) education has imposed on me. When I am no longer afraid of my fears, I will not fall prey to my aggressions, both the outward ones that hurt others and the self-destructive inward ones that hurt myself.

We human beings eschew the path of self-recognition because we sense that our own pitfalls could trip us up. Life is not a wish but also a task. It is life itself that asks questions. Much more than asking life questions, man is being questioned by life. He or she can answer life, can answer to life.

This preceding sentence – is it not an affront? Yes, it is. It is an affront to be confronted. It encourages and urges us not to ask, in a capitalistic, hedonistic way, what our needs and wishes are, but also what duties our fellow human beings impose on us, what life has in store for us. Offending (ourselves) wonderfully translates into offering (ourselves) to act freely and to do what has become necessary.

Maxims of Proximity tries to exhibit visions. Visions are not utopias but instructions for proper, individual actions. This book provides no answers to vital questions. It modestly contains possible signposts or clues, which show the paths we can tread on our own.

The wonders of this world come into existence only because we are doing something unusual, something extraordinary. What did your life mean, you may ask me. I was elected to a dream job and governed successfully. But my homework was left undone. I no longer had time to investigate questions of meaning because I had chilled my soul and anesthetized myself with vain activities – and all the time under the pretense of public service.

The break-up of a relationship of several decades and its ensuing mournful work have substantially influenced the way I think. Emotions went on a roller coaster ride; despair and ecstasy came hand in hand. The pain of loss helped me mature. My weakness in life was to have given too little *proximity*. At the same time I wanted to exercise power over others because I was powerless myself.

The more I am occupied, professionally and privately, with my fellow human beings and the development of their as well as my own motivations, together with the wholeness of humanity and of human personality, the more I grow in the hope of a better life. I am particularly amazed because the generation of my parents (I was born in 1941) rarely exuded positive thinking.

The people of our time would suffer much less if only they had a grasp of a life more fulfilled. The reason for inappropriate social intercourse is a destructive attitude. We have left behind a century in which the limitations and great divides of mankind became blatantly obvious.

To be sure, we need to engage in a critical dialogue with our own failures; however, we also need to turn to positive things. In the law of creation, you can only truly develop when you and others believe in yourself and when you manage to pave the earthly road with hope. A supportive household for children and confidence-inspiring friends for teens are its prerequisites. They encourage us to trace and excavate in our hearts the buried power of *proximity* – to share it, to pass it on, to give it as a gift.

»Somehow bridging the time between two orgasms« – that, as I recently read in a magazine, cannot be the one and only meaning of life, can it? People who focus on the dark side of life charge themselves, like a battery, with negativity. They, as goes without saying, become un-happy.

I want to achieve happiness and do something about it – the origin of this book. Its content challenges me. Do not expect any universal recipes for well-being, because every one of you is unique. But this book drops hints, gives impulses, provokes reflections, offers considerations for a new view of being. We cannot prolong our life; we can only deepen it.

Questions of meaning foster our humanity and require that we put into practice what we consider to be meaningful. In *Maxims of Proximity,* too. If we succeed, we will feel better, which has also been my very own experience, when I radiate joy, make peace, and rid myself of conventions. Our stomachs are full, but our hearts scream. Out of the blue I personally experienced that loss and sorrow may engender growth. I needed this painful »heart attack« – otherwise the subtitle, *Impulses for a Fulfilled Life,* would give the lie to me.

In life nothing changes without our consciousness itself naming a cause. If we admit more *proximity,* we will feel more *proximity,* gain more *proximity.* Is this not your most heart-felt wish, too? Otherwise your intuition, your soul would not have led you to my book, would it? When I turn to a fellow being I find fellowship, or *proximity,* and thus break through my own loneliness. We are born human, of course, but we become human only through a journey to the spring of our existence, a march against the stream of our habits, against our laziness, our conformity.

A successful, fulfilled life wants a lively balance of proximity and distance, of autonomy and community, of inside and outside, of I, you, and we. The interchange of discipline and freedom engenders dignity, joy, sense, and sensibility. Man has navigated and explored the globe, so is it not about time to turn inward, to see our fellow human beings holistically? Is it not about time to invest in not only body and heart alone but also in our souls, in *proximity*?

I wish each and every one of you, my dear readers, the necessary and enduring strength for your very own path. Where there is a goal there is power. Energy and insight elicit evolution and progress of our inner self. Total self-negation is an unreal myth. Deep down in our souls we are creatures of intercourse. By means of you, man becomes I – Martin Buber reminds us. *Proximity* makes our souls melodious. *Proximity* is the real ecology of life.

That this grace pursue you, be with you everyday, is the aim of this book. Let *Maxims of Proximity* heighten your responsibility for your happiness in life. If so, I feel confident that we all will feel better.

Sincerely,

Fred Endres

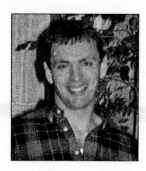

Translator's Preface

Heraclitus says that all things give way and nothing remains.

Walter Pater, 1839–1894

Translating this book has been an abundance of joy and exultation. What fireworks of words and emotions! Because of our proximity, both spiritual and emotional, Fred Endres and I, his translating proxy, have been closely collaborating, using the momentum of the Moment. Like any translation, this one both enriches and impoverishes the original. Like any translation, this one stands only in proximity to its original. However, unlike any other translation, this one is a personal maxim, exclusively added to this American edition.

Translation (Übersetzung). Its etymology, Latin »transferre,« captivates the core of Fred Endres' maxims. Translating means to carry something out into the world, to heave something across, to show past something, to direct something, to uproot something, to entrust something, to metamorphose something, to shift something in time, to apply something, and so forth. The German word adds yet another subtlety: to ferry across a body of water or an abyss – and what else is Fred Endres, the veritable ferryman of proximity, doing in his book? *Maxims of Proximity* is the bridge to the twenty-first century.

All of his maxims coalesce in this translation, in an effort to approximate a fulfilled meaning. May this translation give way to your own »translation« and always remain in translating proximity. May it be an impulse for a fulfilled translation.

Translation is chemistry. Let us translate proximity into love. Oscar Wilde's aphorism sums it all up: »To love oneself is the beginning of a life-long romance.« Finally, I am proud to acknowledge the love and help, for both this translation and my life, of Cecil, Karin, and Rita.

Sincerely,

Professor Nikolai Endres, Ph.D.
University of the Ozarks

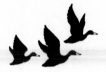

Geniality is nothing but the ability to be amazed.

Georges Buffon, 1707–1788

Amazement

The beginning of all knowledge is amazement. People who are able to be amazed are alive. I can feel joy spontaneously and be amazed at the unexpected, the undeserved, the unfathomable.

The ability to be amazed is one of the most effective stimulants for our immune system. Therefore, I will do everything to invigorate this virtue in me. I will feel more deeply. I will ferret out the secret in/of me.

The development of personality is the most titillating adventure of life. Your willingness to be amazed lets you perform miracles. You are no longer fettered by prejudices. You are following the impulse of the Moment. You are living your dreams instead of dreaming your life.

Consequently, you do not feel depressed when none or only a few of your dreams have become reality. You are poor only when you have never had the chance to dream. Life knows no absolute perfection, only amazing grace. And that is good.

People are more interesting than their public conduct and socially sanctioned emotions, though. Rainer Maria Rilke conceded: Do not forget that life is a piece of splendor. How do we translate this idea? A person who is able to be amazed is able to kiss, to caress life.

Every morning is
a new vocation.

Martin Buber, 1878–1965

Beginning

Let us begin every day with a crucial liberating idea that promises proximity, with forgiving. Consequently, our weaknesses will no longer present obstacles to accepting ourselves and others. Thus the light of joy can reach us.

Every day we also begin with a thanksgiving. We give thanks that we are needed, that people have been entrusted to us, that each and every one makes the world go round with his or her contribution.

Every day is a new beginning. Every day is special, unrepeatable, irrecoverable, and takes its unique course. We give our best because our best enriches us. From the best we derive strength and the apex of our abilities.

We no longer waste a morning with negative thoughts, which impede our personal development and professional output. Every affirmative thought brings a new creative force.

Let us never cease to start anew. Every beginning represents a fountain of eternal youth in an era replete with sadness.

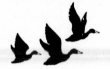

We are what we do repeatedly.
Pre-eminence, therefore, is not
an action but a habit.

Aristotle, 384–322 BCE

Charisma

Our charisma influences the reactions of our fellow human beings. We attract like-minded people, which is one of the great cosmic laws. People with vital energy are bolder, readier to take risks. They burn fewer calories and never burn out.

The women and men to whom people are entrusted carry a particular responsibility. Some move and shake a lot but effect little. These people show off their supposed work ethic like a monstrance, always for their own veneration.

In contrast, there are people with charisma, who have the guts to follow their own inclinations and instincts. They adore others. They foster confidence through acceptance. They further by going farther.

The truly excellent achieve, before their professional triumph, the victory over themselves. With a great deal of self-discipline they are servants who carry out a fascinating task: successfully guiding people. They are virtuosos of emotional intelligence.

So may come what come may.
As long as you live, for me it is day.
And when to go out into the world it is time,
Your home, wherever it is, is also mine.
When I see your visage of lovely light,
Of future's shade I do not catch sight.

Theodor Storm, 1817–1888

Confidence

How come that among our contemporaries we meet so many necrophiles and so few biophiles? Because our calmness and composure have deserted us.

Without composure our daily design loses its perspective. Without composure our ability to differentiate between what is momentous and what is secondary becomes faulty.

The mother of reliability is composure. It estimates the feasible, the reasonable, the chargeable, the practicable. Without composure the art of setting priorities, in both the professional and the private worlds, gets lost.

The composure of the heart confers on life and work an inexhaustible impetus. Inner freedom is the composure of a strong soul.

Such an unburdened spirit reveals self-confidence's graciousness. It is sovereignty. It is superiority in the inferiority of a dilemma.

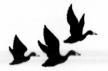

War is the father of all things. Real civil argument(ation) is the mother of a good relationship.

Heraclitus, 544–483 BCE

Contrasts

There will never be happiness for people who exclude sadness and grief from their existence, which is structured around polarizing binarisms.

A society unwilling to suffer neglects the pain we need for human growth and intercourse. We can experience happiness, joy, and confidence only when we survive separation, fear, and sorrow.

We accept our feelings and reflect on them until we improve. This is not anything we do by repressing or merely positive thinking but by mourning and processing.

Conflicts point to deficits and trigger change. They are messages that steer us into the direction of interior dialogue and reflection. They exhort us to deviate from trodden paths and take the road less traveled.

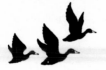

Prudence is suitable for maintaining what one owns. But only courage knows how to acquire.

Frederick the Great, 1712–1786

Courage

As a fearless person you enhance your environment. Intrepidity is uncommonly infectious. It gives courage to people you like, people like you.

With courage you multiply your quality of life exponentially. Amiability is based on your courage and forestalls resignation. Courage is always aware of alternatives and knows how to deal with self-doubt.

Undaunted people are decision-loving optimists. Courageous people show affection without pondering how a partner will respond to it. They delight in the existence of free people because they are at ease.

Courageous people are happy-go-lucky without sacrificing depth. They have found their inner core. They treat themselves to their environment and fellow human beings.

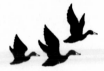

Civilization is a movement and not a condition, a voyage and not a harbor.

Arnold Toynbee, 1889–1975

Creativity

Creative people are curious. They are able to be overwhelmed. They want new modes of life and love the openness of thought. Very often they are simultaneously experienced and innocent.

Creative personalities manifest themselves as a mixture of pride and humility. They are sometimes rebellious and always independent. They have a goal and a clear idea of what they want to accomplish and how they are going to accomplish it.

We nurture our ego and supply our co-workers with thoughts of encouragement and words of wisdom. Nothing is more exciting for human beings than to have their ideas taken seriously and ultimately put into effect. We maintain a warm climate of innovation, so that it pays to be creative.

Creativity is a fertile breeding ground, a scaffold for climbing, a life filled with sunshine. This creative force engenders self-joy, self-effacement, and self-sufficiency.

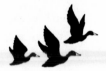

Determination is, in a particular case, an act of courage; but after it becomes a character trait, it is a habit of the soul.

Carl von Clausewitz, 1780–1831

Determination

According to the Christian calendar, we have crossed the threshold of the third millennium. People sensitive to historical time, therefore, have a question that is becoming more and more urgent: Where do we go from here? What are the determining forces that decide how we want to live?

A melancholy look at epochal change will not suffice. Our industrialized nations are suffering from immense roadblocks to political reform. Continuous political congestion is, however, a sign of mental congestion.

Determination shatters the belief that in our enlightened society virtues such as goodness, generosity, openness, honesty, and emotional competence are characteristics of failure. On the contrary, determination empowers us to live these virtues out.

Who wants to advance society cannot live in its center only. Ethical determination is a matter of the inner attitude to the things and people surrounding us.

People ready to act derive their vitality from hidden roots. They treat themselves well and are capable of proximity. They are self-assured. In their souls they no longer serve only to meet rules and requirements. They do more than what is due.

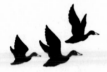

The most wonderful gift to man is joy.

Marquis de Vauvenargues, 1715–1747

Emotions

My soul is breathing again.

Having finally arrived.
Having risked the leap.
Sea, wind, horizon.

Range. Distance.

The sun on my skin.
That is what freedom feels like.
The hectic and nervous life is the Other.

Being with myself.

Loving someone means
To remain always true to yourself.
That is the congruence of proximity and depth.

Grasping. Changing. Moving.

With my soul to new ideas.
With my heart to new tasks.
With joy to everyday life.

Nature. Conscious. Knowing. Being.

Tranquility in a vast valley.
Quietness in the expectation of new sensations.
Knowing that life is more than work.

My soul is breathing again.

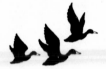

Our head is round so that our mind can change its direction.

Francis Picabia, 1879–1953

Empathy

We are the authors of others. We are inextricably responsible for the facial expressions of others. With these two sentences Max Frisch wishes for human and humane empathy.

Empathy dares to re-discover, in between all the paradoxes and absurdities of everyday life, in between the euphorias and disappointments of existence, something worthy of the name »proximity«: whether the values by which we live on a daily basis are still adequate replies to the frigidity of our society.

Re-evaluating life necessarily provokes us to come clean in head and heart. Without the risk to reflect on traditional patterns and circumstances, our complacent, lazy mind will not allow change. The very challenge, the very coming-out of our century demands this readiness to empathize.

When we empathize and choose love, the darkness of this world will become splendidly radiant. Empathy will help all our relationships, and thus peace (of mind) can spread. Empathy is the conditio sine qua non in every relationship.

Enthusiasm is communicable

Consultant & Trainer for
Employee motivation
Leadership
Public relations

Dipl.-Verwaltungswirt

Alfred Endres

Mayor retired

D-88353 Kisslegg im Allgäu
Falkenstraße 8
 07563/2200
07563/7040

Enthusiasm

Enthusiasm is the opposite of resignation. Without proper exigencies, life becomes boring. Without enthusiasm we cannot arrive at life. Enthusiasm is the stellar path to joy, friends, good neighbors, and charity.

The real secret of success of someone in a position of power and leadership, of everyone, is enthusiasm. This word is derived from Greek »entheos,« someone who has a god in him. You can train it; you can sustain it; you can make it come alive.

Love of life is the only way to master life. Love is always a great chunk of enthusiasm. Let us enter, without hesitation, the El Dorado of this world, especially after defeat and setbacks. Life always has new dreams in store when old ones disappear.

From now on, let us never begin a day without enthusiasm! This enthusiasm will positively infect the people we love and are in charge of.

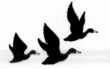

There is no automatic harmony between two individuals. It needs to be conquered and re-conquered in saying goodbye.

Simone de Beauvoir, 1908–1986

Farewell

Why do we cling to images of ourselves, to the expectations of others, without remembering that there is a time for everything? It is important to realize that we are allowed to enjoy but that we also need to say goodbye.

We need to let people go who have left us, in death or in life, for other partners. We can hang on to them in our minds, in our hatred. But that makes us prisoners and keeps us from embarking on a new life, from faring well.

A farewell is also a call to our self-esteem. The future, in every way, is wide open. A younger generation is growing up. It wants a responsibility which, very often, it defines in other terms.

The force and dynamics of life stand their test in letting go, in emphasizing the essentials of life. When we say goodbye, we gain the freedom to create anew. Pain will subside. That is the ecology of life.

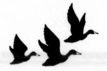

I draw my daring boldness from my sincerity.

George Sand, 1804—1876

Fidelity

Why do so many of us want to be faithful to each other? To be faithful to a person, a thing, or an attitude stems from the basic human need to live symbiotically.

Fidelity is a necessary form of respect. It is the confession that a partner is someone extraordinary, because people have a tendency toward maximum perfection.

Fidelity guarantees that two partners are sharing something special. Thus they can relax and do not constantly have to prove something. As a result, intimate familiarity thrives through emotional security and fulfilled sexuality.

Acknowledgement gives confirmation. Respect offers validation. Fidelity honors the needs, values, and rights of a partner. Fidelity applies to itself the same standards it applies to others. Fidelity encompasses malleability and perseveres in the fickleness of life.

In order to sustain a relationship we need to learn to respect our differences. When a man and a woman (or other partnerships) become too similar, in the long run their attraction for each other wears off. To keep fidelity alive, differences must be cherished. This tenet inaugurates the chance of a lifetime: growing closer to each other, with each other, and for each other.

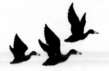

Living means changing oneself.
Being perfect means having
changed a lot.

John Henry Newman, 1801–1890

Forgiveness

Forgiveness is the disarming of a hard heart. For-giving is giving for love. A human being must be capable of forgiveness. Because of our fallibility we know how motivating and powerful forgiveness is.

Instead of chastising ourselves and feeling guilty, we forgive ourselves and the people we encounter. Thus we eliminate bitterness, which is the clotted disappointment we do not want to combat any longer.

Forgiveness becomes vital energy when we are dumping dead weight and opening ourselves to a better future. Forgiveness is asceticism, a simpler life for the purpose of a better life.

How much forgiveness does one need?
As much as one needs love.
And how much does one receive?
As much as one loves.

Love me, when I merit it the least, because that is when I need it the most. That is my cry for help and hope in you!

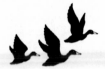

Liberty means responsibility. That is why most men dread it.

George Bernard Shaw, 1856–1950

Freedom

How often do we catch ourselves surreptitiously longing to be free and fly like a bird? And how little do we do for it, although as individuals we have a right to the rainbow of difference and diversity.

I hope for a chance, not an assurance. I do not want to be a citizen on welfare, who is being taken care of because the public is responsible for me. I have to embrace risk. I want to yearn for something in order to put it into practice. I want to be a visionary.

I would rather cope with the impending difficulties of existence than lead a quiet life. I am in search of sense, not safety or security. I want to achieve success and therefore will survive any shipwreck.

Very often, too often, we waste our longings. We content ourselves with the remembrance of a body handicapped with fear. Why are we so caught and caught up? Why can we not fancy hope?

Breaking free from a cliché takes a lifetime. Because of affirming myself I have learned to think individually and act authentically. In this way I became free. When I am internally free and live out this freedom, I am more loveable.

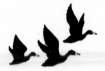

Friends are gardens in which one can rest and relax.

Antoine de Saint-Exupéry, 1900–1944

Friendship

Friendship is the art of freedom. Thus Albert Camus begins his Song of Solomon. It is not profit or fun but intrinsic value that determines friendship. There is indeed love at first sight, but hardly ever friendship. It must grow and mature; it must be cherished and constantly renewed.

Friendship leads me out of narrowness and gives me proximity. I will no longer get lost in myself. I will rather open myself up, pay attention, become resourceful. When I enter the private sphere of my significant other, I will make myself at home. Friendship makes me carefully conscious of how others feel and how they change. A person becomes a friend when I feel that he or she has been entrusted to me, and that I can trust him or her.

Let us make time for our friends. They will become an unheard-of spring of happiness. They will inaugurate new opportunities for understanding and levity. Let us be thankful for fellow human beings who (have) become faithful and sincere friends. Profound friendship makes our existence really worth living.

A person is a person only insofar as he or she is capable of friendship. Deep friendship is grace, is redemption. Friendship at its most precious has no need for explanations.

Fulfilled love is the most excellent source of joy.

Thomas Aquinas, 1225–1274

Fulfillment

A lot of us have let the love of life slip away, some even unnoticeably. Yes, we do suffer a lot, but most of us do so quite comfortably.

Fulfillment will always be directed at evolution. It is development for the sake of transition, and transition for the sake of completion.

We gain fulfillment from never-ending creativity. Never is fulfillment a matter of age, education, or origin. It does not need the crutches of wealth and unceasing validation. No, it is simply an affair of the heart.

Let us face the future with open hands and minds and cast off all burdens. A life fulfilled is levity, a piece of freedom. Through your vitality you orchestrate all kinds of possibilities for growth and maturity.

A fulfilled life aspires to utopias. It encourages us in the contradictions of everyday life. It comforts us in the attractions and addictions of existence. Fulfillment is full of hope, in this life and beyond.

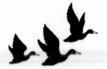

Nothing has ever been conquered entirely. Everything must be fought and re-fought for every day. Otherwise it gets lost.

Romain Rolland, 1866–1944

Future

Time is not just transitoriness, endless drifting. It races to the finish line. And that only is what gives time its brunt, its tangible impetus. That indeed bestows on the future its ultimate seriousness.

You develop visions for the people entrusted to you. You try to anticipate the change in values. The salient feature of your activities is humanitarianism and touching warmth.

Joint responsibility cannot arise in the realm of over-bearing, where people selfishly indulge in the conviction that success cannot be shared. Not blasphemous self-doubts of a plaintive time but an optimism ready for action makes the future shine bright.

Acting in fond hope for the future gravely calls on us to account for our personal belief and our common hope.

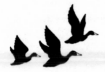

Those endowed with gratitude are also gifted for joy.

Zenta Maurina, 1897–1978

Gratitude

Gratitude is proximity expressed in words. At the same time it is joy echoing joy, another happiness for the happiness of others.

Grateful people give others the power for goodness. Gratitude is giving, is sharing, is a maxim of love. Gratitude is a secondary delight which prolongs a primary one.

There is nothing people long for more than the selfless gratitude of others. Let us be grateful that we are needed. Can we feel empathy for what it is like for a fellow human being who is no longer needed in the job market?

You are grateful for everything that enriches your life. With such an inner attitude you encourage your partner, colleagues, and co-workers. You motivate by showing gratitude.

Gratitude is the secret of friendship.
Gratitude is the memory of the heart.
Gratitude is the measure of our lovability.

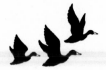

Supreme happiness in life is the assured knowledge to be loved.

Victor Hugo, 1802–1885

Happiness

Happiness puts the crown on a self-confident personality. Who starts out in search of happiness commits to a life-long game. He or she is no longer a distant spectator but, in the thick of it, its very protagonist.

Picturing and imagining our longings often obscures happiness. A victory over ourselves, trifling as it may be, is worth a thousand times more than the delight we take in some hero's vicarious victory.

Admittedly, this piece of advice is tricky. But once you have decided to believe, first and foremost, in yourself rather than in others, you will gradually but solemnly rise above the doubts that obstruct necessary change. You can raise your standards because your happiness does not depend on sheer luck anymore but on your own tiny steps that, worked on every day, will become giant leaps.

Happiness is the basic longing of man. The gates to happiness eventually open to the outside, not to the inside where I am content with myself and myself only. Being capable of happiness is always tantamount to being worthy of happiness. Happy the soul that is friends with itself.

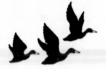

I want to be loved or I want to be comprehended. That is one and the same.

Bettina von Arnim, 1785–1859

Harmony

For millennia, people have been searching for meaning. Doing good and making others successful stabilizes my own psychological balance. This ethical and moral foundation gives me harmony.

When I look after inner harmony, I will live in peace with myself and my environment. When the winds of change are blowing, some build walls, others, the clever ones, windmills. When I catch and channel this wind into a challenge for different impulses, as an initiative for motivation, I will, when all is said and done, bless myself with abundant harmony.

Life can be incredibly wonderful, when I am in possession of my inner core. Then I am helpful and give joy. Then I perceive goodness in every creature. New harmony is thus re-generated.

Through my goodness I prop up confidence in life. There is no dwelling without people who transmit harmony. They offer me a home, intimacy, and security.

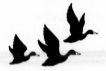

More beautiful than utter wealth is
the expectation of hope.

Emanuel Geibel, 1815–1884

Hope

People who love human beings will always put their hopes in them. Hope is not the expectation of a happy ending but the conviction that everything has its meaning and makes sense, whatever its outcome may be.

My own hope for man's inherent goodness has very rarely been disappointed. When as a leader I imbued my partners with confidence, they thanked me by in turn confiding in me.

Only people who put themselves out and are ready to assume responsibility create hope. Lamentation and resignation make one guilty, by association, of the misery of reality, which, in any case, is always in the eye of the beholder.

Hope that shuns risk is no hope at all. Hope, by definition, believes in the adventure of love, of proximity, of happiness. It dares to jump into the marvelous, the unknown.

Hope is the prerequisite for being and development. Never surrender your hope in the goodness of human beings, of co-workers, of partners. Start with it today. People with hope manage to cope!

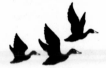

It is hospitality's deepest meaning
to lend a helping hand to someone
on his way to his eternal home.

Romano Guardini, 1885–1968

Hospitality

We human beings are and always will be on the road. We know how lonely, how fragile the stranger and guest can be. Therefore, we constantly need hospitality on this planet. We need to rely on the kindness of strangers. It is not a question of education or riches but the plain readiness to approach someone else.

Hospitality is not anything we learn in school but simply an attitude of openness, of being-together, of spontaneous cordiality. Being face to face with someone, we recognize this person as our sister and brother. We have a presentiment of their immense, ineffable longing for warmth.

The Greeks are our models. They put the stranger under the protection of the god Xenios. »Xenos« in Greek means guest *and* stranger. Any export-oriented nation should welcome strangers in order to approximate the Greek ideal. Hospitality defeats xenophobia

At a banquet my homesickness expresses a yearning for security. The joy of passing on food and information instigates the hope of having been accepted and taken in. Hospitality is proximity and completion.

Every human being needs other human beings to become more human. Hospitality freely given comforts someone near or next to me, someone who, in our egocentric, cold society, often shivers. I shall not simply defend the »I« but also cherish the »you.«

The civilization of peace begins with hospitality.

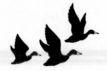

The legacy of an age lies not only in
its harvest but also in what it sowed.

Ludwig Börne, 1786–1837

Humanity

A society that has forgotten how to exhale, that only rapaciously swallows, avariciously piles up, onerously toils, and carouses like gluttons, loses its compassionate humanity. It misses charity and thus its happiness.

Humanity and positive thinking belong together. They are tolerance lived. They admit mistakes and enhance themselves through partnerships.

Humanity also gives others a chance. People who keep pushing themselves into the center of the universe will fall prey to attrition. They will not become (more) popular. The power and dynamism of life consist in letting go.

Humanity's twin is humor, which is superiority even in the inferiority of embarrassment. Humorous people will not be derailed by a setback.

A human(e) frame of mind is a fundamental and profound interest in our existence, even in a flawed world.

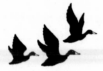

The most generous people are usually the humblest ones.

René Descartes, 1596–1650

Humility

The knowledge of mortality makes me become humble. I am a creature of beginnings and endings. However, I do have to make decisions here and now. This choice is a question of upbringing, culture, and ethical maturity.

Stupidity reveals itself in a lack of humility. At the beginning of the twenty-first century we have lost a lot of humility. We are convinced that virtually everything can be done. But I am not allowed to pursue everything I like, neither in my environment nor in my pleasures.

The more often I satisfy a desire without gratitude or love, the less joy I feel. All happiness without humility wears out, in particular the more intensely I search for it. I experience more profound happiness when from time to time I have to forego it.

Humility is always a question of character, which is formed in the stream of life and human growth. It is won in a struggle with innate traits. I experience humility and character not as a gift of creation but as a victory over myself.

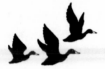

Tell him only, but tell him modestly, that his love is my life. The joyful feeling of both of us will be his proximity to me.

Marianne von Willemer, 1787–1860

Joy

All this shall become dazzling joy:

Questions that open up new paths.
Thoughts that provoke innovations.
Reflections that do not conceive of existing things as
    unchangeable.
Ad-ventures that create more openness to the world.

Let us look forward to this day,
Because it is our life,
The life of all life.

In its course is all
Reality of existence:
The joy of growing,
The magnificence of doing,
The glory of creation.

Because yesterday is nothing but a dream
And tomorrow only a vision.
Today, lived with joy,
Turns yesterday into bliss
And tomorrow into hope.

Therefore we look forward to this day.
Whoever strives for the impossible
Faces no competition.

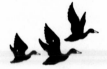

The richer one is in judgement, the poorer one is in prejudices.

Henry Miller, 1891–1980

Judgement

We too rashly (pre)judge the people we encounter. Everybody has his or her lovely characteristics too, which we should not devalue through prejudices or negative first impressions.

Low self-esteem, self-deception, judgementalism, prejudice: they are classic examples of fallible errors in judgement. They open the door to dangerous manipulation of others.

Having a low opinion of others often subconsciously includes a dose of self-hatred, which is a projection onto others of our own lack of self-esteem. Errors in judgement carry the seed of self-destruction.

Let us live in harmony and love of ourselves and our environment. The willingness to do good for others – real good will and benevolence – will enrich us and make us truly fortunate.

We delight in someone else's success. This joy keeps us youthful in a destructive age. In conclusion, this ethical and moral canon will, more than any judgement or opinion or verdict or sentence or decree or ordeal or award or appraisal, bless our society with peace.

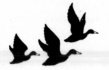

The future disturbs us; the past holds us captive; therefore, the present escapes us.

Gustave Flaubert, 1821–1880

Life

We human beings have been created for life; therefore, we are responsible for the here and now. The most important day of our existence is today and everyday. When I neglect the present, I hinder life. I miss out when I strive for the ultimate security guarantee. Life, not life insurance.

Anticipation is more frightening than experience. The fear of tomorrow always comes a day too early. Replenish life with meaning, for then you will ameliorate the lives of others, too. You do not wait for life; you let it happen. When you look too far ahead, you make life a torture and agony.

The sins of omission, it seems, are the only ones that will not be forgiven. Continuously change the rhythm you are accustomed to. Thus you are enjoying life, leisure, pleasure, the favor of the Moment. The contradictions of existence are alleviated by the therapy of trust.

Life has exquisite benefits. It is a joy to be alive! With this epicurean essential you will no longer comprehend life as a morass of self-impediment, of spoiled opportunities. Rather, you will retain the subtle sensitivity to breaches of trust, to the hypocritical mendacity of bourgeois morality and complacent cant of middle-class culture. Thus you imbue life with more meaning and plenitude.

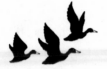

People who love themselves and each other display the god living in them.

Carl Rogers, 1902–1987

Love

For centuries, ethics has been haunted by a question: Can loving be learned? My answer is: Yes, because in every human being love is a deeply implanted force. Yet it does not work autonomously. Love is essentially, like freedom, neither a reflex nor an instinct.

Every declaration of love is an affirmation of presence and the present. It can never be an insurance policy for all future. It is the promise for openness and the effort to live up to my partner's expectations. Wanting from him or her everything that life has to offer is hubristic. Nonetheless, everybody needs other people in order to be more than a body.

What is love? Is it agape, is it caritas, is it eros? Underdeveloped love follows this tenet: I love because I am being loved. Mature love knows: I am being loved because I love. Immature love objects: I love you because I need you. Sincere love proclaims: I need you because I love you.

Love is a voluntary gift; therefore, it cannot stand exclusiveness. Love knows no perfection. Like so many animate things it has its limits and limitations. However, people who accept the universe less than whole-heartedly love not even half-heartedly; they love not at all. The only way to master life is to love it.

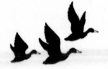

Let it never happen that after you meet someone, he or she is not happier.

Mother Teresa, 1910–1998

Meeting

Our talking to others makes us human, Karl Jaspers reveals. A person completes and perfects himself or herself not just as an individual. He or she can grow only in meeting other people. We are all creatures of social intercourse; therefore, we need to approach others.

In our total devotion to the you, we accomplish unconditional and unselfish openness. In patient dialogue we reap the stars of love from the sky. Light comes into existence where we meet:

Hearing	instead of simply listening
Understanding	instead of standing around
Respecting	instead of despising
Laughing	instead of deriding
Questioning	instead of answering
Trusting	instead of doubting
Giving	instead of taking
Meeting	instead of confronting.

With every consciously-lived meeting, heaven is extending to earth and earth is becoming heaven.

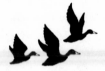

The mastery of the Moment is the mastery of life.

Marie von Ebner-Eschenbach,
1830–1916

Moment

The interchange between eros and psyche, between sexuality and soul, triggers lust. Thus the Moment becomes a physical, mental, and emotional opportunity for various choices: cuddling, pillow-talking, praising, admiring, enjoying, amazing, warming, whispering sweet nothings.

Lust can heal – when we put this force to a loving use – whatever we decide to do with the Moment or intend to give our partner. Lust eradicates our doubts and feelings of inferiority.

Let us practice more the joy of the Moment,
Giving ourselves spontaneously,
Yet also ecstatically,
Occasionally even orgasmically,
Excitingly, relaxingly,
With the knowledge that with our feelings we fulfill a
    part of creation's mandate.

A letter can be a spontaneous aphrodisiac. Soothing green, gushing winds, bitter cold, the warming sun, a chilling rain, or a purifying thunderstorm yield comfort and security.

What luck, when we, unfettered from so-called inevitable constraints, enjoy the Moment. People will find their happiness reflected in their own smiles. Then the Moment has become a monument to light.

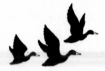

We composers are the projectors of the infinite into the finite.

Edvard Grieg, 1843–1907

Music

Andrzey Szczypiorski, the Polish Literature Prize-laureate, has defined music as the most exquisite nourishment for the heart. For him, music, in a class of its own, is like a beautiful woman: seductive, mysterious. He loves her, he covets her, but he fails to recognize her …

The gift of human proximity does not offer itself in all stages of our life. Creation grants other internal forces to console us. One of these wonderful presents is music. What motivating fascination it reveals!

In addition to its healing and invigorating power over the psyche, music, especially as a cultural experience, significantly contributes to our physical, mental, and social well-being. Music sustains our emotional growth and spreads peace.

Music, in the paradoxes and absurdities and in the dis-illusions and illusions of everyday life, dares to caress our soul with a soothing balm. Music is the nourishment of proximity, and love the nourishment of music.

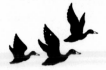

The gift of love cannot be given. It waits to be accepted openly.

Rabindranath Tagore, 1861–1941

Openness

At the core of every mature relationship is mutual space. It really indicates an appreciation when a partner occasionally does not understand us.

Leave your partner time to cope with conflict. Do not intrude too early. Intimacy grows from openness. Severing ties unites more than any coercion.

The quality of our relationships reflects personality. What we perceive as a problem today may be a solution tomorrow. Knowledge comes about through the path of openness, of dialogue.

Openness creates an atmosphere in which we arrive at a better understanding of ourselves, the necessary prerequisite for full development. An open person is not afraid of emotional tempests, of fireworks of love, of maybe even a rhapsody in blues.

To shed dependencies and to be open to people and things around us is true life and sparkling vitality.

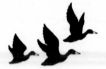

First you do what is necessary, then what is possible, and finally you will be able to do the impossible.

Francis of Assisi, 1181–1226

Optimism

An optimist (from the Latin root for »the best«) sees in every difficulty a possibility. A pessimist sees in every possibility a difficulty. Affirming the world means to say »yes« to the earth the way it is.

With this attitude I am no longer really troubled by things to come, for when I overproject into the future, my existence becomes a burden to me. I believe in life and drink it to the brim.

Optimism produces a scintillating life in all its shades. It rescues us from insipid mediocrity. A time full of contradictions needs people whose everyday vitality radiates hope.

Optimists walk on clouds, the same clouds under which pessimists gloomily have the blues. For the optimist, life is not a problem but a solution. He or she is susceptible to the preciousness of the Moment.

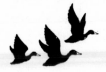

I can because I want what I have to do.

Immanuel Kant, 1724–1804

Passion

Who possesses passion is alive. Acting passionately means serving a cause with devotion. If you do not want to play an intellectual game, you choose charitable action – as a vested personal interest in the destiny of a fellow human being.

Passion is converted into energy, into responsibility for people entrusted to us. A decisive psychological component of responsibility is the need to pay attention and use perspective. We let realities, compressed internally, make an impression on us.

This world is run by people who contribute more than their duty because the sum total of egos still makes no whole, certainly no common weal. There is no life without passion.

Nobody can void the interchange between soma and psyche, between body and soul, because man was cast holistically. The stimulants of the soul such as anger, wrath, sadness, guilt, or longing we often dismiss as life-threatening. However, whoever rejects passion suffocates.

In the passion for the whole the ecstasy of creation is mirrored. Acting passionately yields a life fulfilled in a world too full.

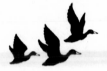

We could never learn to be brave and patient if there were only joy in the world.

Helen Keller, 1880–1968

Patience

Nobody has a monopoly on truth. We are practicing patience when in an argument we remain open(minded) to the more persuasive point. This intellectual integrity is contagious.

Patiently I try to live the day without wanting to comprehend life in its totality. I give in, but I do not give up. Thus I am acting with humility and will accomplish more.

Patience is not self-debasement because it has good intentions. When I remain patient, I facilitate and convey proximity. This trait makes patience so human and gives it a winning streak.

We humans are no puppets of our genes. Free will lets us grow and mature, when we practice patience. Then life will bless us with plenitude, radiance, and love.

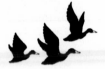

The most important thing is not to think a lot but to love a lot and to act in a way that excites love.

Teresa of Avila, 1515–1582

Prayer

Do you still find the tranquility, the relaxation, and the sense to pray? Many of us will answer in the negative. But there is energy in this »no.« Such restlessness shows that everything you have suffered, lived, and believed did indeed shatter your view of things.

It is also self-consciousness. Praying actually means to get in touch with yourself before God. I myself at least strongly believe that this world never ceases to have miracles in store for those of us who affirm and love life.

Wonderful creation,
I thank you,
Because there is a human being
Who loves me.

He opens himself to me,
She takes me in,
He looks at me,
She listens to me,
He talks to me,
She is there for me.

I am happy
Because – once again – there is a human being
Whom I can love
As much as I am capable of loving.

The more complete someone is, the more respectfully he treats others.

Thomas More, 1477–1535

Respect

Respect recognizes a partner's needs, values, and rights. We must give him or her the same importance we attach to ourselves. Respect is the most precious and onerous task of love. When I love someone I am respectful; I am also respectful for my partner's sake.

Our self-definition culminates in the commitment to the principles of human rights. This commitment translates into being careful, paying attention, keeping an eye on the other, taking him seriously, honoring her, and respecting the other for who and what he or she is.

Respect as the appreciation of the people entrusted to us includes cozy security, which makes room for self-development and self-control. Respect encourages a kinder, more amiable being-together.

When I have internalized respect for every creature, I know that people are gifts, temporal donations to me. A dear partner is our greatest gift. No one has a claim to the other. Who wants to possess the other cannot escape a terrible tangle and disrespectful deception.

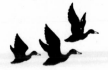

We are responsible not only for what we do but also for what we do not do.

Jean-Baptiste Molière, 1622–1673

Responsibility

Responsibility is the courage to be an exemplary model. It is curiosity rather than satiety. Consequently, we may not twist the truth and brush aside facts; we must perform tasks and avail ourselves of opportunities; we must seize the potential and power we have.

Exploring what is within reach,
Not only listening to voices that tell us to stop.
Demolishing borders,
Overcoming prejudices.

Responsibility involves tolerance and openness to everything colorful and creative. Do not look away; go ahead. Leave the fringes and margins of rumor and insinuation; blow fresh air into the world. Whet your appetite for change; become a part of the future of us all.

The key to a successful relationship lies in both partners' taking responsibility. That is the opposite of victimization.

Victims think that they are not to blame for what happened to them or for how they feel. They often suppress their anger and clandestine resentment instead of eliminating this burden in mutual com-munication.

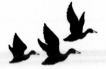

Life can be understood only backwards. But it must be lived forwards.

Søren Kierkegaard, 1813–1855

Self-Reliance

We have no complexes; complexes have us. The difficult relationships from infancy through adulthood to our later life result in complexes which are often repressed.

How can we respect ourselves when people have failed to give us (enough) respect? How can we love ourselves when love has been allocated to us only as a service in return for good conduct?

However, we can learn to deal with our deficits to such an extent that they no longer impede our progress in life. Terminating self-accusations from the inside makes for self-reliance. You are self-confident when you trust your standards, when you admit your inadequacies, when you are able to take a stand for yourself and others.

Over and over again we need the audacity to risk scandal, which impresses and furthers our self-confidence. From the art of self-love emanates self-confidence. It is a foundation of vivaciousness and proves the will to life.

The fear of the »you« betrays a lack of self-reliance. I do not search; I only find. What Pablo Picasso clothes in this epigram shall be your programmatic lighthouse: Tackle life self-confidently!

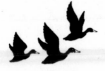

I was searching for god but did not find him. I was searching for myself but did not find myself either. I was searching for my fellow beings and found – all three.

The Talmud

Solidarity

We should not look on the misery of the world as mute or silenced spectators. Everyday we are summoned to be activists for solidarity. Solidarity is the quintessence of civilization, the authoritative impulse for ethical acts.

Not everything that befalls us happens without cause and effect. Causes and effects stem from a sense of solidarity, which should direct our actions. Security and proximity require hope-making solidarity.

So many souls nowadays transmit SOS. The more freely we live, the higher the stakes of solidarity have become. Solidarity and self-accountability come hand in hand. Solidarity is at home in a society with a social conscience, a society that assumes responsibility for the individual.

The survival of the earth depends on the insight that everything exists, not autonomously, but synergistically. Practicing solidarity means sharing. It gives friendship, neighborship, partnership, and any form of community a future.

Solidarity augments and advances. It helps and hydrates. It allies and advocates. It binds people together and allows them to endure shock. It enriches my life and extends my mind. The cultivation of solidarity begins in human hearts.

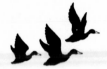

The stars of our happiness lie in ourselves.

Heinrich Heine, 1797–1856

Spontaneity

Spontaneity means being able to do what you long for at a certain Moment. You are surprising yourself because from the routine of your everyday life you pluck out-of-the-ordinary joy.

You have the courage to follow your intuitions. You become spontaneous and extemporaneous because you are sure of yourself. Then you will also see that problems exist in order to be solved by means of further self-improvement. Let us regard problems as a potential for growth.

Moments in which we allow spontaneity remain unforgettable. You are living flexibly but not rashly and impulsively. You are casting off the so-called constraint of having to follow a predestined life-style. You are bidding farewell to opinions that distort the here and now.

I am confident that creation has put us in the place where, according to its great scheme of things, we belong. Progress is and remains the challenge to materialize utopias through spontaneity.

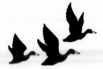

Real charity is more than the power of sympathy. It is the ability for affection.

Martin Luther King, 1929–1968

Sympathy

As long as we are fair-weather people, we lack proximity. When we develop compassion we are responding to love, even if our partner is lost in his or her mood swings.

Sympathy is your interest in someone else's fortune. The term is derived from Greek »sympatheia,« the willingness to partake of suffering, to be com-passionate. We encounter sympathy in devotion, affection, kindness, mercy, and generosity.

Compassion is sharing other peoples' suffering. It is indeed religion, a re-connection and re-conciliation with the Creator, a reincarnation of God. Sympathy enables us to do so many things that pure reason alone cannot bring about.

Compassion is deeply embedded in our moral values. Compassion sympathizes with everything that suffers. A smile is a light flashing up in your eyes, which the Greeks regarded as the window of the soul. When we feel compassionate, all the lights are on and somebody *is* home.

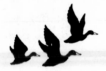

When you look at me, I am sitting in the sun.

Fyodor Dostoevsky, 1821–1881

Tenderness

Everything in life starts with thoughts. Tender thoughts are powerful stimulants. Self-satisfaction is self-squandering. You are competing with others instead of tenderly giving yourself to others. You are losing yourself instead of finding proximity. You are practicing dominant authorship instead of comradeship.

In this world so many things happen serendipitously, without obvious meaning; yet nothing is meaningless. Everything has its intrinsic value, even when I may not (yet) emotionally or rationally recognize it. Tenderness is always meaningful because in it we discover humanity.

When I am willing to be tender, I ask myself in the evening into whose heart I brought light today. Tenderness never runs out of breath; it is never breathless. It is the diligent care for our own life. It cannot be exercised without self-love and charity.

Tenderness is a declaration of compassion. It starts with the ability to listen and ends with the willingness to listen. It is empathy and means approaching and approximating the other.

Sisterhood and brotherhood always express tender devotion to the degree of self-effacement. Tenderness is the essence of the joy of all creation. It is the ultimate measure of our ability to love and be loved.

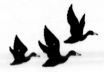

All human errors are impatience.

Franz Kafka, 1883–1924

Time

I pray for power and proportion, so that I will not be rushing through life but sensibly plan my day. I will focus on rays of hope, silver linings, and my zenith. And at least off and on, I will also find time for a cultural delight. Such was Antoine de Saint-Exupéry's view of his time-management.

Seizing the day means to subsist moment after moment, Moment after Moment, and wholly sucking in life. Then we will no longer have to lament or dread our everyday omissions.

You know what is really important in this world. In your professional realm as well as in your private life you set targets and priorities. Every day you take time for yourself. You do not postpone life. You try to simplify your life and clear it of rubbish.

Thus you are consciously scheduling hours for lingering, dreaming, being silent, looking, forgiving, being amazed, reading. What matters to you is the quality of time or quality-time, not the quantity of time, mere dissipation. More time for more space.

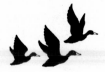

Trust is the greatest self-sacrifice.

Friedrich Hebbel, 1813–1863

Trust

Trust is devotion. Who trusts surrenders. Without trust every society, every partnership is doomed to fail. Trust people, so that they in turn will trust you. Nothing is, in effect, more motivating.

Trust is the firm belief in the ability, integrity, reliability, and seriousness of our partner. Without trust we fail to live up to someone's intentions. Trust also means that for every irritation, for every offense there must be a plausible explanation.

Instead of believing in life we are sowing distrust when we want to be in control of everything. In order to develop trust in our own capabilities we need to multiply confidence. Advancing trust in life is the best precaution.

When we are trustful, we attract the secret powers of humanity. Inadequacies recall the finity and evanescence of life. What keeps us going is in no way our own attainments — but indubitably trust.

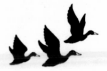

Every human being is created and born for the sake of another human being.

Martin Luther, 1483–1546

Unselfishness

Unselfishness can move mountains and stir hearts.

Responsibility without unselfishness makes one unscru-
pulous.
Justice without unselfishness makes one hard.

Truth without unselfishness makes one intolerant.
Education without unselfishness makes one ambivalent.

Intelligence without unselfishness makes one cunning.
Order without unselfishness makes one petty.

Expertise without unselfishness makes one arrogant.
Power without unselfishness makes one violent.

Possession without unselfishness makes one stingy.
Belief without unselfishness makes one fanatic.

Why do we live, if in this millennium we do not become
less selfish for the common good?

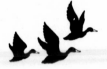

Impossible? One thinks: a lot is. Yet when the time has come, one does the impossible because there is no other way.

Gwen Bristow, 1903–1980

Vision

Visions are no utopias but instructions for action. Without visions we repeatedly catch ourselves feeling self-pity. This in turn restricts our faculty for happiness.

Without visions we remain trapped in sadness, constantly feeling our pulse, as Martin Luther points out. Without visions we practice nothing but self-immolation.

The quality of our goals determines the quality of our future. Before every objective there is a vision. It is not a dream but the first step to action. Visions orient us and make us grow wings; visions excite and emancipate.

Building visions equals thinking the unthinkable. Nowhere will anything good or prodigious evolve if it has not been promulgated by responsible heads and hearts.

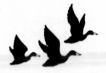

It is in human nature to think rationally and act illogically.

Anatole France, 1844–1924

Vulnerability

Vigilant and constructive people engage in conflict. What would happen if we stopped striving frantically and obsessively for harmony? We may trust that everything appropriate for us is, in any case, just waiting to be found.

We are doing a budding relationship a disservice when we busily emulate the golden calf of a life without conflict. Openness, on the other hand, helps you get a date. Halfheartedness avoids the contact we all long for. It promotes lack of commitment and self-loathing, the conviction that we cannot stand ourselves.

Rather, show more vulnerability. Thus you grow emotionally and personally. You are embarking on a lucrative exploration into your innerness. You are treading the uncharted territory of your authentic feelings.

Each and every one of us is born with the potential for self-love and vulnerability. Consequently, we are able to love others, but also to criticize others. And only thus may we leave ourselves, fearlessly and vulnerably, to love's devices. Then we are in conscious charge of our lives yet remain sensitive and vulnerable to partners and fellow human beings alike.

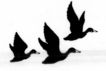

The world is so empty when one imagines only mountains, rivers, and cities in it. But to know that occasionally there is someone who harmonizes with us, and with whom we tacitly continue to exist, only that makes this terrestrial globe an inhabited garden.

Johann Wolfgang von Goethe,
1749–1832

Warmth

What would we human beings be like without emotions? We have a right to them. A life without them would be quite inconceivable. Without our emotions in full swing, our existence would be numb, worthless, null and void.

The plenitude of life must involve more than rough and tough reality. The commonplace becomes life only when it also includes the unexpected, the undeserved gift. It is better to err in life or in love than to run away from love because of the fear of warmth or of making mistakes.

We are always in motion, doing something. Why then (for a change) do I not do anything to do nothing? My overstrained psyche needs chicken soup time and again. A creative pause is cathartic and helps to cleanse. The soul functions and suffers according to the same principles as our physical organs.

Without warmth our calendars get more crammed and our relationships emptier. The less time I waste on small talk, the more time I have for people who need me, who matter to me. Nouvelle cuisine instead of fast food.

At the same time it is inherent in mankind not to be profound all the time. Only with this thought in mind do we derive warmth and proximity.

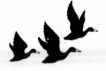

Choose as your companions for the orbit of life: Those who broaden the horizon of your heart and mind. Those who encourage you, who divert you, who hasten with you heavenwards.

Friedrich Schiller, 1759–1805

Well-Being

Our personal growth reflects the trinity of attitude, faith, and perception. Faith sustains your everyday rituals, which in turn reinforce faith.

Let us expect something good from every day. In our actions we try to visualize the well-being of all humanity. Is our faith just dry, artificial flowers instead of an airy, fragrant bouquet?

Religious salvation, when it indifferently dismisses the dramas of secular history, annihilates security and well-being.

When we cultivate this train of thought, an inner feeling of well-being will develop. The conviction that every human being has his or her intrinsic value inspires it. Therefore, every human being merits esteem, not intolerance.

Let us trust this well-being. If so, we will internalize, more than skin-deep, the raptures of creation. It is the fire sent by God!

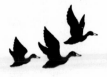

Youth is perpetual intoxication. It is the fever of reason.

François de La Rochefoucauld, 1613–1680

Youth

Youth always has something to do with lovability. I cannot love this person or that person, only love and life, Hermann Hesse indulgently proposes.

Being young means so many things: to retain the daring for marvels, to be amazed at an iridescent glow in everyday life, to dare something completely new, to quench the thirst for the impalpable, to levitate on the lightness of tomorrow.

Youth is ready to embrace the imagination, the fantastic. It opposes adventurousness to procrastination and ardor to convenience. Youth, never jaded, distrusts probabilities of one hundred percent.

We are young so long as our heart heeds the message of courage, seizes the grandeur and power of the day, comprehends the infinity the world, and thrives on the excitement of the unknown.

Youth is not a caesura in life. It is a state of the soul.

The World Needs More Proximity

Life succeeds according to a plan that first of all we need to search for and find deep in our souls. This book contains fifty-two (weekly) sketches and inducements for experiencing more *proximity* – in relationships, in friendships, in the professional domain. It has no patented claim to comprehensivity, because there simply is no blueprint for compassionate humanitarianism anyway.

Yet it is a secret of meaningful, supportive relationships that from time to time we adorn the rhythm of everyday life with climactic, ecstatic spirits. To exactly such a wonder of the world *Maxims of Proximity* wants to stimulate you, excite you, encourage you. It wants to put forth impulses for the mastery of the mystery of life.

It all goes back to giving *proximity* a chance, so that it can ripen and spread. Not only in our dreams but also right in our hearts. Thus *proximity* can pave its way to our fellow human beings – and to you, too.

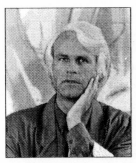

Fred Endres, born 1941, graduated from university with a diploma in administration. After official missions in Berlin and in Bonn for the Federal Department of Economic Cooperation and Development, he was mayor in the German state of Baden-Württemberg for sixteen years. The father of two children, a college lecturer, and the author of several books currently works as a management consultant for motivation and tourism in, among other countries, the Ukraine and Belarus.

Life succeeds according to a plan that first of all we need to search for and find deep in our souls. This book contains fifty-two (weekly) sketches and inducements for experiencing more *proximity* – in relationships, in friendships, in the professional domain. It has no patented claim to comprehensivity, because there simply is no blueprint for compassionate humanitarianism anyway.

Yet it is a secret of meaningful, supportive relationships that from time to time we adorn the rhythm of everyday life with climactic, ecstatic spirits. To exactly such a wonder of the world *Maxims of Proximity* wants to stimulate you, excite you, encourage you. It wants to put forth impulses for the mastery of the mystery of life.

This book is written for people who consider durable relationships neither an accident nor a matter of sheer luck, but rather willed and lived creations of human *proximity*.

It all goes back to giving *proximity* a chance, so that it can ripen and spread. Not only in our dreams but also right in our hearts. Thus *proximity* can pave its way to our fellow human beings – and to you, too.

Printed in the United States
41609LVS00002B/9